Losing Weight to Gain Control

Loving Your Weight Maintenance Journey

By Gwen S. Alexander

TABLE OF CONTENTS

PREFACE

The title of the book represents the way I started feeling as I lost weight. I've lost 70 pounds and several inches off of my body. As I lost the weight, I began to feel that I was gaining control of my weight and my life.

The book itself started as a guide for me to follow. Each chapter represents lessons I learned on my way to living in weight maintenance. I hope the lessons I learned can be of help to you also.

ACKNOWLEDGEMENTS

I want to thank my Lord and Saviour, Jesus Christ, for not giving up on me when I was ready to give up on myself. I also want to thank my family and friends that encouraged me during the process of writing this book. I also want to thank Jade Simmons and Dr. Fred Jones for lighting a fire under me to take action and get this book written.

DISCLAIMER

The information in this book is for informational purposes only. This book is not meant to be used, nor should it be used, to diagnose or treat any medical condition. The author is not a medical or health professional. Please seek advice from your doctor or medical professional before beginning any weight loss program.

All motivational quotes in this book are that of the author unless otherwise noted.

INTRODUCTION

A journey can be defined as traveling from one place to another. What do you do before you go on a journey? You plan how you will get to your destination and what supplies you will need to get there. The same things you do to prepare for a journey are the same things you do to lose weight and keep it off. Many of us have tried following roadmaps for diet programs that were made by others that didn't fit into our lifestyle. These programs can be very restrictive of what foods you eat or may require large amounts of time for exercise. I want to help you begin your journey and map the route you will take to lose the weight and keep it off. Journeys aren't always a straight path. There are turns in the road, hills to go up and down and sometimes you have to stop to refuel. When you reach your destination, you realize those turns and hilly roads were what made the journey eventful. Let's get started mapping your journey.

Motivational Quote

Don't be afraid to take the first step to begin your journey.

GIRDLES AND WEIGHT LOSS

"If you wear a girdle you won't gain weight!" This is what my grandmother told me when I was a child. If you don't know what a girdle is, think of Spanx in the shape of a panty. From first grade to seventh grade I wore girdles to keep my weight under control. Every day my stomach hurt because I wore girdles that were too tight. The foods I ate as a child were frozen pizzas, potted meat in a can, Vienna sausages and anything fried in a lot of grease. My family didn't realize my weight gain was due to the poor food choices we made. I was told I ate too much but was never taught what healthy food and portion sizes were. Even though I knew I wasn't eating well, I did not control the food that was brought into the house.

Unfortunately my unhealthy eating habits continued into adulthood. One of my low points with food happened in high school. I had my first job when I was a senior in high school so I had money to start buying my own

10

food. One day I went to Burger King and ordered two Whoppers with cheese and two large fries. I didn't order any soda because I didn't want the workers to know that was for me, ALL OF IT! I went home and closed my bedroom door, ate the food and started to cry. I didn't realize then that I was an emotional eater. I ate to numb any negative feelings I had.

When I went to college my weight continued to increase. I was wearing a women's size twenty six which was the largest size you could buy at any clothing store in the early 1990's. In 1996 I decided to lose one hundred pounds in a year and I did! The only problem was I wasn't happy and always felt I needed to lose more weight to be happy. Then I started to restrict my calories to the point I was eating 1,000 calories or less a day. I didn't realize how dangerous it was to eat so little. Everyone told me how good I looked but on the inside I was so miserable. I was able to keep the weight off for about three years but it was a struggle to control my weight. Eventually, I gave up the fight and proceeded to gain the one hundred pounds back. Many times between the year 2000 and 2010 I tried to lose the weight again only to regain the weight I'd lost. I tried the caloric restriction plan which had worked before but it wasn't working now. I asked myself what am I doing wrong this time?

Then in July of 2011, I went through another low point in my life. One day when I got home from work, I was waiting for my dinner to warm up in the microwave. While it was warming up, I just started stuffing myself with cookies, peanut butter and any leftover food I had. Then I ate two large servings of the food I had just prepared. I remember feeling very full and tired. I sat in my La-Z-Boy chair and started to cry just like in high school all those years earlier. I didn't know why I ate all of that food. I realized in that moment I have to stop abusing myself with food. By December of that year, I started again with trying to lose the weight. This time was going to be different though. The difference was I didn't care how long it would take or what changes I had to make in my life.

Have you had a low point in your life related to your weight? What's your motivation for wanting to do whatever it takes to lose the weight and keep it off? Every person who has gone on a diet is a success. They have successfully lost the weight. Where many of those diets fail is they are not sustainable for a lifetime to keep the weight off. This book will guide you through making a plan customized for you.

Motivational Quote
When you have challenging moments, don't quit. Keep pressing through them!

RETHINK THE WORD "DIET"

When I hear the word diet restrictive eating comes to mind. That means no desserts, no breads, no pastas or any other foods that are supposed to be off limits to lose weight. Are you willing to never go to parties because the food there is off your plan? Wouldn't it be nice to know you can eat a slice of cake and not be off your eating plan? There are diet plans that say eat fruit then some plans say fruit is bad. Some diet plans tell you to stay away from a whole group of foods. Telling yourself you will never eat a particular food again or stay away from social gatherings is not realistic. Here's a new phrase to use instead of diet – weight maintenance plan.

Have you ever heard of the story of the tortoise and the hare? In the story the hare and the tortoise have a race. One would assume the hare would win because he can move faster than the tortoise. The story ends with the tortoise winning, not the hare. Do you know why the tortoise won the race? The tortoise won the race because he was consistent. That is what your goal will be for your plan. Don't make yourself feel bad if one meal you eat is not the best choice or your whole eating plan was bad for that day. Remember, all food can fit into your plan.

Motivational Quote

The tortoise beat the hare because he was consistent not because he was the fastest.

MAPPING YOUR JOURNEY

Get out a piece of paper or your computer. I want you to make a list of weight loss plans you have followed in the past. After you have made your list, write down which parts of the plan you followed were good and which parts may have been extreme in a negative way. An extreme thing I did in my first attempt at weight loss was expect my body to survive on very little food. The next question to ask yourself is why did you stop following the plan? When you realize what parts of the plan weren't sustainable for you, don't do them this time. Trying harder at a particular weight loss plan will not make it work if it didn't work before.

Many plans have one good thing in common, they make you conscious of what you eat. Look at your list and highlight the parts you could do the rest of your life. Something I noticed when I made my list of my first attempt at weight loss was I had more free time. In my life now, I work a full time job, have a side job and that's not counting all my other responsibilities. I do not have hours to dedicate to focusing on my plan. This time I had to be realistic about the pace my weight loss would take. Are you willing for it to take you six months to lose ten pounds? What about five years to lose one hundred pounds? Being realistic about your time frame to lose the weight will keep you motivated. Read over your list when you are tempted to do the same thing as before as a reminder that this time, you will do things differently.

After you've made your list it's time to weigh and measure yourself. Oh no, here we go. You can start by measuring around your waist, hips, upper arms and anywhere else you want to track. Why do you want body measurements? Sometimes during your journey to maintenance you will lose inches on your body while the scale is not moving. Several times during my journey the scale was not moving but I was losing inches on my body. This is another way to keep you motivated throughout the process.

The scale is a tool for you to use to gage where you are. Think of it as a compass that is showing you what direction you are going. Do not make the number on the scale the focus of your journey. Let me repeat, do not make the number on the scale your focus. I do not recommend weighing every day because your weight will fluctuate daily. I have read articles about people that lost weight and weighed themselves daily. This is not necessarily bad but what happened with some of the persons is the scale began to dictate their mood for the day. I've noticed by weighing once a week, it gives me an overall idea of how my eating habits are affecting the number on the scale. This allows me to focus on habits I need to change during the week. On the piece of paper you logged your weight loss attempts in the past, write the date, your starting weight and measurements. Now you know where you are starting so you can see how far you will go on your journey.

Motivational Quote

Decide to make the necessary changes in your life to lose and keep the weight off.

TRACKING YOUR FOOD

The first thing I did when I lost one hundred pounds several years ago was throw away all the food in the refrigerator. I stopped all cookies, had one cup of soda a day and cooked everything I ate. I even gave up eating at restaurants. I did all of this in the first month. This was a radical plan for me. Little did I realize I was setting myself up for failure because this was an unrealistic way to live the rest of my life. What I did this time in my journey was not as drastic. I started to become conscious of the portion sizes of the food I was eating. I bought an inexpensive paper notebook from a local store to log my food. There are also apps you can download on your smartphone to help you keep track of your food. I wouldn't worry about tracking calories or other nutritional information just yet. You want to write down what you ate and how much of it you ate. When you see the information staring you in the face it will keep you accountable. You'll also want to buy a set of measuring cups, measuring spoons and a food scale. Almost everything you buy in the store has a nutrition label on it. If you look at the label it will tell you what a serving size of the food is – either how many cups or ounces. When or if you eat breakfast, write down how many cups of cereal you poured in your bowl. How many eggs did you eat that morning? Be honest, your body knows what you ate even if you didn't write it down. Did you go to a fast food restaurant for any of your meals? Even if you ate two packs of M&M's, write it down. Next time, your goal would be to eat only one pack instead of two. Then the next goal would be to ask yourself, what's a better snack alternative? If your car was on empty would you expect it to go when you put your foot on the gas pedal? Why would you expect your body to perform without any fuel in it? Log your food for at least a month so you have something to look over to see if there are any patterns you need to change. Do you notice you eat more food in the evening? Do you notice you snack all day and then eat a huge meal at night? When you realize what you're eating, then you can modify your behavior.

Motivational Quote

Don't expect your body to run on empty.

IT MATTERS WHAT YOU DRINK

Liquid calories make a difference in your plan. You will need to write down what you drink because your body does count those calories. If you are a coffee drinker, the sugar and creamer you put in it has calories. Do you like sports drinks? Many of those have lots of calories especially if you drink larger sizes. Frozen coffee drinks are loaded with them also. When logging your liquid calories write down how many cups or ounces you drank. The label on the bottle will have the information of how much is in it.

Water is the main liquid I drink. The other liquid calories I drink are hot chocolate, tea, soymilk and orange juice. I don't drink each of these every day. The rule I made for myself is I can have one or two beverages besides water a day. That includes anything from the list you just read. Anything you drink can fit in your plan, just make sure you track what you are drinking.

You can take a week or several weeks to get into the habit of tracking your food and drink. Take it slow and give yourself time to adjust to the new habits you are learning.

Motivational Quote
Remind yourself liquid calories matter on your weight plan.

START MOVING

You don't have to do extreme exercises to get started. If you haven't been physically active, trying to do an hour of exercise won't be easy. Besides, if you don't enjoy the exercise you are doing, why do it? When I started on my journey I did what I had done in the past, exercising like crazy for an hour. This time on my journey I didn't have the money to pay for a gym membership. The times when the gym was open didn't work for me anyway. My decision was to workout in my home and take walks as the weather permitted. The DVD workouts I started with were The Biggest Loser or any other workout like those. I thought every workout had to be long and hard so I burned out pretty quickly on exercise. I was not going to give up because I knew I needed to be active. I discovered on YouTube you can search for any duration and type of exercise. There are indoor walking plans, cardio exercises and weight training available for free. This meant I had to plan my workouts and get any equipment if needed. I didn't have a lot of money to spend on equipment so I did body weight exercises. If you're not able to do the exercise, modify the movement. Many of the videos have someone that is doing a modification of the exercises. You may be saying to yourself, that's great for you Gwen, but I have no idea where to start. I don't even know what I like! I recommend you start with walking; walk in place for five minutes, walk outside-JUST GET MOVING. If your mobility is limited, start with just walking across your room in your home. There are also exercises that can be done sitting if you can't stand. Once you build up your endurance you may want to try low impact cardio workouts with some sculpting with weights involved. You can buy a set of two, three or five pound dumbbells to use.   If you don't have thirty minutes to dedicate to exercise, try breaking it into fifteen minute increments. The goal is to move and get active. I do advise you check with your doctor before beginning an exercise program.

If you have invested in weights, keep them in a place where you see them all the time. I keep my workout equipment next to my television. If I'm watching something on television, I pick them up and do some exercises while the show is playing. You can go online or to your local library to check out books on exercises you can do to workout with weights. There are websites that will give you a plan based on what type of exercises you want to do. Do a search for "upper body workouts with weights." You can search for "lower body workouts." Working out with weights will help tone your body. The goal is to make the time to exercise.

Maybe the gym or classes at the gym would work better for you. If you decide to become a member of a gym, ask if you can have a session with a trainer. Make sure the trainer understands what your goals are. Taking a group exercise class may be better for you. This will hold you accountable since other people are involved. If you know you have paid for the class and it's scheduled, you are more likely to keep going. I go to classes at my local gym when my schedule allows it. I enjoy talking to others that are trying to get healthy and live a better life. I have learned I prefer home workouts, but that could change in the future like many journey's do. Here are some tips to help you find ways to add physical activity to your life:

1. Schedule it. If you schedule it, you will do it.

2. Have your workout clothes ready for the next day.

3. Have your workout planned. If it's a walk, have it already written down as your activity for the day. If it's a weight training session, have your exercises written down.

4. If you have a job that involves sitting all day, stand up and move when possible.

5. After dinner, instead of sitting to watch television, take a ten minute walk. Walk five minutes, turn around, and walk home. You many find once you get moving, you'll keep going.

Motivational Quote
Make the time to fit exercise into your life.

QUALITY FOOD

Now that you're in the habit of writing down what you eat it's time to focus on the quality of your food. You may have heard the term "clean eating" thrown around a lot. Every person seems to have their own definition of what this means. My definition of clean eating is finding better food substitutes for ones that may not be healthy for you. Here is an example of a food substitution I did. One of my weaknesses is peanut butter and chocolate. To be more exact Reese's Peanut Butter Cups are my weakness. Do you know in two of those peanut butter cups there are 250 calories? I stopped eating them because they weren't worth wasting my calories on. I wanted to get more food for my calories. I want to introduce you to something that made a difference with my food choices. When I started my journey I was eating 1,500 calories a day. I was tired and in a bad mood much of the day. I did lose some weight but hated the way I felt. I thought to myself this way worked before, why isn't it working now?

One day I was listening to a podcast called Fat2FitRadio. (As of this time, they are not recording new episodes.) The hosts were talking about eating your BMR. I thought what in the world is a BMR? It's your Basal Metabolic Rate. Your BMR is the minimum amount of calories you need to exist. By exist I mean if the only activity you did was lay in bed all day. You can go online and do a search for BMR calculators to find what your BMR is. The one I used asked for your height, your gender, age and weight. When I put in the information it asked for, I couldn't believe what I saw. According to this calculator, I should have been eating almost 2,400 calories for my activity level. I didn't think the calculator was right. I decided to go ahead and raise my calories in small increments to see what would happen. As my caloric intake increased, I noticed I wasn't hungry or tired. Write down your recommended caloric intake in the front of your food journal. That way you always know what your goal calorie intake is. As you lose weight, go back to the BMR calculator and put in your numbers again. The reason for doing this is the amount of calories you need will change as you get smaller. I noticed as I lost weight I didn't want to eat as much. When I input my updated information, the chart showed my caloric intake was less than when I initially started.

At every meal I have ½ cup or 1 cup of a vegetable, a side dish, some type of fruit and four to six ounces of a meat or fish. A few examples of my side dishes are brown rice, mashed cauliflower, or a salad. Desserts are also a part of my eating plan. The desserts I make are usually single servings. If the dessert recipe makes several servings, I put them in individual containers for later. Snacking once or twice a day has also helped me stay on track. My snacks are 200 calories or less. Some of the foods I snack on are Greek yogurt, hummus and fruit. You may want to use this as a guide to figure out what foods will work for you. Remember, you need to enjoy what you're eating or you will not continue on your plan.

I am not against frozen dinners, canned foods or any type of prepackaged food. I did notice a difference in the way I felt when I started to cook my food and use better ingredients. Makeover recipes are a great way to continue to eat foods you love. There are websites, cookbooks and magazines dedicated to making your favorite recipes healthier. Remember my peanut butter chocolate addiction? I found a recipe for an individual peanut butter chocolate cake using powdered peanut butter. It fills two roles by giving me more food for my calories and it tastes great. If you like fried chicken, did you know you can oven fry your chicken? If you like French fries make your own. It is a lot of work but as you find recipes you like and learn shortcuts in the kitchen, your preparation time will be less. Here are some suggestions to help you make your eating plan:

1. Find makeover recipes of your favorite foods. If you are looking for them on the internet, read the reviews of others to see how they liked it.

2. Sit down one day a week and plan your meals for that week.

3. Try to buy whole grain pastas, breads and lean meats.

4. Use measuring cups, spoons and a food scale to measure the portions of your food.

5. When eating out, avoid foods on the menu with phrases like creamy, fried, and smothered in. Ask if the food can be prepared differently than what the menu lists.

Motivational Quote
Think of food as fuel for your body.

THE RULE OF 80/20

Trying to eat perfectly 100% of the time is not realistic. I've read articles that recommend you follow the 80/20 rule for weight management. The 80/20 rule says 80% of the time to stay focused on eating right and 20% of the time don't worry about what you are eating. Personally I follow a 90/10 rule. Why am I so strict on myself? The reason is my past performance with food. At the end of the week I review my food journal to look for patterns in my eating habits. I noticed when I went off of my food plan, it took three days to get my eating habits under control. This happened every time I went off my plan. I made a decision based on my past performance that I have to be conscious 90% of the time of what I am eating. Take the time to review your food journal. Do you notice patterns in your eating habits when you eat certain types of food?

Something else I did differently on my journey was remove the words "cheat day" from my vocabulary. When I reviewed my food journal I realized on my cheat days I was eating way too much. I was undoing all the work that had been done during the week because I ate so much on my cheat day. I began to think of my cheat day as a day I consume more calories than usual. I still ate quality food but on that day I would have larger portion sizes of my meals. When I changed my way of thinking of a cheat day I didn't want to overeat. When you are having your 20% eating day, don't try to eat as much as possible. Enjoy what you are eating but remember if you want more food, you can have it.

You've made it this far so pat yourself on the back. You've been logging your food and getting physically active. If you haven't started any of this yet, still pat yourself on the back for wanting to do your weight loss differently this time.

The next chapters have nothing to do with food or exercise but they are key in helping you maintain your weight once you lose it. This journey is not just about hitting a number on the scale or looking good in clothes. It's about doing a life makeover as well. Looking good in your new clothes is a nice perk though.

Motivational Quote

Find a way to accomplish your goal.
No excuses!

WHAT'S YOUR MOTIVATION?

Pantyhose! You may be thinking what does pantyhose have to do with motivation? My motivation when I started this journey in 2011 was pantyhose. The plus size pantyhose were sold two in a box and the other sizes were sold three in a box. Both sizes were the same price but I was only getting two with the plus size pantyhose. I'm a shopper that wants the most for my money and wanted the three pack of the pantyhose. My motivation has changed over the past few years. My motivation went from pantyhose, to wearing smaller clothing to never wanting to feel like I did in July of 2011. Ask yourself, what is your motivation? I've heard many reasons from others what their motivation is for wanting to lose the weight. A few reasons I've heard are to be a better parent or make someone they respect proud of them. These are great for wanting to lose the weight and keep it off. Ultimately your motivation should be because you love yourself and want to take care of yourself. I realized at the start of my journey I needed to do this because I loved myself enough to take care of me. Realize you are worth taking the time to take the steps necessary to get healthy. Your motivation will help you make better food choices. It will motivate you to stay on your plan when you feel you are ready to quit.

Motivational Quote
Remind yourself daily why you're doing this.

THERE ISN'T ENOUGH TIME

There never seems to be enough time in the day. What I have learned is some of us are deliberate about how we use our time. How much television do you watch a day? How much time do you spend on social media? Other activities you could do with that time are plan your meals and workouts for the week. Sunday is the day I plan my meals and workouts. It makes my week less stressful when I have those planned. My nightly routine involves relaxing around eight thirty at night and by nine it's bedtime. I've figured out my best time to exercise is in the morning. I am not a morning person by any means. My past experience has taught me when I saved my workout for the evening, it usually didn't happen. Something more important always needed to be done at the end of the day. I did something radical and started getting up at five o'clock in the morning. I never knew anyone could function at that time. I decided to make exercise a priority and planned accordingly. You will have to begin being deliberate with scheduling your day.

In order to free some of the hours of your day, you may have to say the word no. Practice saying this word several times a day. No! You may have to say no to family members to make the time you need to focus on your life. I'm not saying don't ever say yes to anything. If there is an event you really want to go to, then go to it. Don't just say yes to everybody to make them happy. Remember, you will never make everyone happy. Take the time to take care of yourself.

Motivational Quote
Everyone has 24 hours in a day. How will you use your 24 hours?

RESTFUL SLEEP MATTERS

You need sleep. Let me say it this way, you need restful sleep. A restful night's sleep helps the body repair itself. Think of the last time you slept soundly and how you felt the next morning. You probably felt recharged and ready to start your day. Have you noticed when you're tired you seem to eat more? The types of foods your body wants are the ones that will give you a quick boost of energy. The quick energy boosters are candy bars, doughnuts, cookies and soda. The problem is once the sugar high is over then you are tired again. Then the cycle repeats itself, eat sugar, feel awake, sugar level drops, feel tired. Here are some suggestions to try and get a good night's sleep:

1. Keep noise to a minimum in the room you are sleeping in.

2. Have the room you are sleeping in at a temperature that is comfortable for you.

3. Go to bed at the same time every night and wake up at the same time every morning.

4. Keep electronic use to a minimum before going to bed.

If you're always tired please consult a physician. If you are on medications, there may be side effects that interrupt your sleep. Maybe you have a condition like sleep apnea that causes you to stop breathing periodically through the night. Don't be afraid to ask for help in this area. Getting adequate rest will help you make better food choices throughout the day. You will eat because you are hungry, not because you are tired.

Motivational Quote

Restful sleep is the best way to control hunger while awake.

EMOTIONAL OR PHYSICAL HUNGER?

Some of my friends tell me they overeat because they are bored. I ate because the food was in front of me. You may have your own reasons why you mindlessly eat. Emotional hunger is trying to satisfy an emotional need with food. When you eat your emotions the foods you crave will make you feel worse not better. The foods you want to eat are potato chips, cookies and anything high in calories and fat. The problem with emotional hunger is it will never be satisfied with food. This type of hunger is only satisfied by taking the time to deal with what is bothering you. Did you have an argument with your significant other? Are your children having problems in school or with friends? Is your work situation stressing you out? Any of these events could trigger an eating episode. How many times have you told yourself, I deserve this hot fudge sundae because I worked hard today? You can also use food as a way not to feel any emotions. I used to overeat to suppress any negative emotions. I have never been diagnosed with an eating disorder. I am speaking from what I learned about my eating habits from the past. Anytime I had feelings I didn't want to deal with, I would stuff myself with small amounts of food before I would eat my main meal. I later realized I did this because I didn't want to deal with negative feelings from past or present situations. If you feel you have emotional issues that are more than you can handle, reach out and get help. Talk to a friend, talk to your doctor, or find a professional that specializes in eating disorders. Don't give up on getting the help you need to lose the weight and keep it off. You are worth it.

Motivational Quote
Ask yourself, am I physically hungry or emotionally hungry?

FORMING A SUPPORT TEAM

Having a person or team of people to support you during your journey is very important. There will be times when you want to quit on your plan or on yourself. The people you choose to be on your support team will encourage you to keep going. The people you choose to be on your team doesn't have to be family or friends. The people you find to support you could be in an online community. There are several online communities you can join that have everyone at different stages on their journey. The sad truth is your loved ones may be the ones that are trying to sabotage your efforts. They have seen your past attempts and may say this will be like the other times. Your loved ones may be scared if you lose the weight you will change and not want them around anymore. Let them know how important this is to you and how much you need their support. Be prepared for a negative response from some people you ask for help. I've been told it's not my problem, it's yours. I've also been told why should I change, you're the one that needs to change. Hearing that from the people you care about makes you want to give up before you even start. That's why you need to have the support of people that you can contact during times when you need encouragement. There are online newsletters you can subscribe to that can give you encouragement. The ones I subscribe to are usually weekly newsletters delivered to my email. Many of them give you advice on how to handle situations that happen while you are losing the weight. Have you thought about how to handle negative comments from people? What about dealing with the times when you think you aren't making any progress? Your support team will be there to cheer you on and remind you to keep going.

There will be times when you may not have access to your support team. Be ready to encourage yourself when you don't have access to anyone. Your friends want to help you but they are not with you 24 hours a day. Read your motivational quotes and reread your reasons for taking this journey. This will help you through the times when you think you can't do this anymore. You can do it and you will do it.

Motivational Quote
Tell yourself, I can do this!

TRACKING NON-SCALE VICTORIES

It's wonderful to see the number on the scale go down. There will be times during your journey when the scale will go up or not move at all. It can get discouraging when you put so much work into eating healthy and getting active and nothing seems to be happening. I realized two years into my journey I needed to focus on accomplishments other than weight loss. I started making a list of non-scale victories. Examples of non-scale victories are wearing smaller clothes or running your first 5K. One of my most memorable non-scale victories happened Thanksgiving Day of 2013. I registered to do a one mile walk and it started to snow when all the walkers were at the starting line. I decided even though it was snowing to go ahead and do it. I began to cry while walking because I would have made excuses in the past of why I should not have done this. An added bonus that day was I didn't overeat at Thanksgiving dinner.

That's one of the non-scale victories that keeps me motivated. These victories are important because they help you focus on living life, not just existing. Write your victories down and read them often. Post them on your refrigerator, on the bathroom wall or where you get dressed each day. I recommend logging your victories at least once a week. You will be surprised that the scale may start to move when you put your focus on other aspects of your weight loss journey. Document and celebrate your victories during the journey.

Motivational Quote
You are more than a number on the scale.

START LIVING NOW, NOT LATER

Start living your life to the fullest now.
Don't wait until you reach your goal weight to
enjoy life. Look for opportunities to try
something new every day. Go out and
introduce yourself to someone you don't
know. Go to an event of something you're
interested in. Don't wait until you lose ten
pounds to be sociable or dress better. Start
dressing better at the size you are now.
Losing weight will not make your life better if
you're not making changes to how you live
now. I didn't put my life on hold during my
journey. I was not going to wait until I
reached a certain number on the scale before I
started enjoying my life. I started attending
more events in my community. I would
purposely start conversations with people I
didn't know when I went out. What is it you
have been putting on hold in your life? What
is it you want to do but kept telling yourself
I'll do that when I lose weight? Make a list of
things you want to do that you never felt you
could accomplish. This will also motivate

you to continue with the plan you have made. Go out and get busy creating your awesome life right now.

Motivational Quote

Don't wait until you reach a certain number on the scale to start living your life.

GET INSPIRED

Having a role model is a great way to stay motivated on your journey. Find someone who has lost the amount of weight you want to lose. This can be someone in your family, in your community or online. You can go online and do a search for people that have lost weight and kept it off to help you to stay on course. I have three individuals that I regularly follow for daily motivation to not give up. The reason I chose them are they each had a lot of weight to lose and they lost it slowly. When you find your role model, follow them on social media. Many of them have daily inspirational newsletters you can sign up for that will encourage you.

Something else you will notice as you progress on your journey is you will eventually become someone's inspiration. I've had my friends and people I didn't know ask me how have I lost the weight and kept motivated. Someone stopped me one day to tell me she thought of me when she was exercising that morning. She said to herself if Gwen can do this, so can I! In that moment I was very humbled and shocked. I have spent so much time looking to others for inspiration I never thought anyone would look to me for it. There are people that are watching you to inspire them. Let that be one of your reasons to not quit.

Motivational Quote

One day, you will be someone's inspiration.

GAINING CONTROL

It's amazing how other areas of your life improve when you gain control of your eating habits. You become conscious of habits that you may need to stop in the areas of finance or relationships. Your finances may get better as you learn to stay on a budget. I have done a budget for several years but sometimes wouldn't follow it very well. I began to be consistent with putting my budget into action. Your relationships will begin to improve as you take care of yourself and learn to set boundaries. Find ways to spend extra time with loved ones or doing activities you enjoy.

I also took control of how I invested the hours of my day. I started deciding what activities I needed to put on a hold and which ones to work on right now. Do you have a book you have wanted to read or even write? Start taking control of how you spend your time at work. If you work from home, let everyone know you have office hours. Those are the hours you are working and can't be disturbed except for emergencies. If you work for someone else, analyze the time you are at work. Is there a way to organize your time to be productive in a shorter amount of time? If you aren't deliberate in how you spend your hours, someone else will tell you how to spend them.

Gaining control of your thoughts is something you must do. What you think of yourself is the way you will portray yourself. If you think you'll never be able to keep the weight off, you won't. Start telling yourself you will be successful this time. Train yourself to respond to a negative thought with a positive thought. You'll have to fight to take control of what you allow in your mind. You are worth the fight. The best part of gaining control is you become a participant and not a spectator in your life.

Motivational Quote

Take control of your life and become a participant in it instead of a spectator.

ENJOY THE JOURNEY

There will be times during the journey you will want to turn around and quit. While you are focusing on food, exercise and changing your life, don't forget to enjoy the process. Don't become focused on losing the weight quickly just so you can say I lost all of this weight in a short amount of time. My goal in the beginning was to lose 100 pounds in a year. I had done it before and besides, it sounds impressive to say that. I quickly learned my focus was on the wrong thing and I wasn't enjoying myself. Enjoy that you are making changes in your life not just physically but emotionally also. You are becoming a stronger version of yourself. I wouldn't change anything about my journey. The times the scale number went up or my food choices weren't the best are when I had the most personal growth. During those times I learned I am worth making the changes in my life to be happy. Accept the times when it seems like you aren't making progress. Enjoy learning the lessons that you will be able to teach someone else one day. Work hard and focus, but don't forget to enjoy the process of who you are becoming, the best version of yourself.

Motivational Quote

Reaching your destination is not the prize. The prize is becoming a better version of yourself while taking the journey.

ABOUT THE AUTHOR

Passionate, talented, and dedicated to everything she does, Gwen Alexander is an emerging artist with a lot to offer the world of art and those who appreciate it. For years, she's been writing inspiring articles, encouraging others to stay committed to their dreams and to never give up. A published author with a desire to help people lose weight safely and effectively, she desires nothing more than to come alongside others as a friend and confidant who encourages with positivity and radiance.

As an accomplished pianist with a Bachelor of Music in Piano Performance from Louisiana State University, she has also used her music to influence others. Using her innovative piano storytelling program—Piano Tales—Gwen brings stories to life as she highlights actions with her music. Creative, engaging, and quite a bit of fun for those who would otherwise think of classical music as something to fall asleep to, she's refreshing the way people view and hear the beauty of music. In moving, entertaining ways.

With a great love of writing, history, music, and fashions throughout the ages, Gwen is a theatrical and enthusiastic artist with a desire to connect with others and help them connect to the world around them. A lover of historical reenactments, you can often find her attending and dressing up as someone from days gone by, or you may find her perusing the glossy pages of recipe books and hovering over a stove with a new, exciting meal simmering. Whatever or wherever you find her, though, you'll find her with a soft contentment highlighting every aspect her life.

Life is meant to be lived. Every facet. Every mountain and valley. And for Gwen, this has become a reality she wants to share with others, encouraging them to find their value and use it to better the world around them. One note at a time.

Here's how to connect with Gwen:

Website: thegwenalexander.com

e-mail: thegwenalexander@gmail.com

Facebook: facebook.com/thegwenalexander

Twitter: @TheGwen1685